The *Slay* Academy

8 Weeks to Design the Whole and Healthy
Life You Deserve!

The *Slay* Academy

8 Weeks to Design the Whole and Healthy Life You Deserve!

Monique Holmes

"One simple change can change your life for good." – Coach Mo

I was born and raised in the "South," only to me, it was home. I didn't even consider North Carolina the South; that was more like Alabama and Mississippi, right? Since moving to the "Big City," I realized how southern I am, and my charm is unmatched. We were poor, but I had no idea what that meant. I grew up in the 80s and, growing up in this time, meant you had to be active as a kid. There weren't many cellular phones, personal computers, and (thank God) there was no social media! We had about 30 cable stations max. And I had a few TV shows that I loved, but primarily cartoons in the morning, and then the rest of the day was mine.

Later in my teenage years, the good ole '90s came roaring through, and I grew to love shows like Soul Train, The Fresh Prince of Belair, and Martin. Still, without a digital video recorder (DVR), or on-demand, you had to be in front of the television on time, or that was it. You missed it. Can you imagine not having on-demand? Oh, I cringe at the thought. But, even so, we never let television shows control our lives. There was all sorts of drama going down at my neighborhood park, and that was way better than any TV Show.

There were Double Dutch tournaments, kickball seasons, and football playoffs. We jumped rope, mastered hopscotch, and played hide and seek until one night I was never found. I knew how to hide, I guess. Basketball and dodgeball were two of my favorite sporting games. Though I was tall, I was clumsy and needed too much refining to get on the school basketball team. Of course, organized sports were different from neighborhood games.

My hope for the NBA was looking slim to none. Even with all this activity, we would get bored and make up some new games, choreograph the latest Salt-n-Pepa song, or memorize the Biggie lyrics that I would secretly write down. This practice would later help me in school, as I learned that writing helps with memory in any subject matter. We were crazy active kids.

When the streetlights came on, we would eat, bathe and crash. And some nights, right before I could fall asleep, my mom might burst into my room, "Baby girl...baby girl...hey Moses!" She affectionately nicknamed me Moses, which I adored. Come show us that new dance you and your friends were doing outside." She was way too loud and way too hype. I would sleepily stare at my mother like she was crazy and wonder what time it was. I mean, did she not know we just had a soccer tournament at the park?! "Aww, mommy, I'm tired," I would say while smirking. But mother, the greatest convincer, would say, "It will only take a few minutes, and you are the best dancer in the world, so you need to show off." I loved to dance, and she knew it. "Can I have soda, too?" She would laugh and say, "Anything for my baby girl!" So here I go, off to the living room in my Care Bear nightgown, going to dance for my life. I would dance, and the adults would cheer me on like Beyonce, or Janet Jackson, as we didn't know Bey yet. We rocked hard through the '80s and '90s; if you missed it, ask your parents.

I reminisce on these times because this guide will also help you revisit your childlike innocence through vivid visualization techniques and help you identify any behaviors or triggers that may be hindering your overall health goals. You can find your true self in your inner child, the one with big dreams and no fear. I began to play school sports in middle school. I ran track in the spring, marching band in the fall, and competed in Community track all year round. Thinking back on what I did, all of this sounds insane to me now. But at the time, being active was just normal to me. I was constantly trying to gain weight and build muscle. I had to be about

90lbs of all lean muscle. When you practice and train this much, you can practically eat anything and not gain an ounce. My overall health was excellent because we ate whole and organic foods. These weren't the terms we used, though. I was fortunate enough to have been raised by my Great-Grandmother. She mainly cooked veggies from her garden, rarely from a can, and most food items that were in a box or bag were not allowed in the house. That's right, Grand-Ma Sue Bell often rejected donation boxes.

Sheesh, I was so upset because my metabolism was shooting through the roof, "Can we please have that box of pancake mix at least?" Afterwhile, Granny let us have any of the donated food; she was a sucker for the grandkids. We were what I call "food poor" at times. It was weird to understand because sometimes our house had all the food and, sometimes, we didn't have any food. I can vividly remember when we did not have food, and I could feel the hunger pangs eating at my back. This skinny little kid would be starving. So, I would make butter sandwiches and syrup sandwiches if I had to. Despite many obstacles, we were prideful people, and we weren't asking for help. We would have to wait. I never went hungry for too long, but it was long enough to create a traumatic pattern in my life. Fear and anxiety about food began to settle in my mind. As soon as we got food, I would overeat. I would load my plate up. I'm talking two hot dogs, two burgers, all the sides, and then I'd get up and get another plate. I would eat until my stomach hurt and was hard as a rock.

I thought that this food could last in my stomach in case the food ran out again. I heard people say things like, "Where is she putting all that food?" and "No one is feeding that child." However, I could eat all the food, and no one would ever stop me. All of it! Because I was slender, no one noticed the problem or even cared. But if I were thick, someone probably would have stopped me from eating all that FOOD!! I created a traumatic relationship with food that I will spend the rest of my life fighting. But it is so worth the fight. Fight for yourself, your children, and all those around you who are watching and rooting for you to win. Many family members, and even friends, would call me greedy. I just agreed that I was greedy and hungry all the time. "Hey, look, Mo will eat anything, ha ha ha," friends and family would all chime in. This cycle of events repeated throughout my childhood and caused an eating disorder.

I began to disassemble this thought pattern after reading a book called *The Four Agreements* by Don Miguel Ruiz, which you will find in the recommended reading section. The author talks about those early childhood years when we begin to form impressions about ourselves. Family and friends make statements, consciously or unconsciously, that trigger us to believe these thoughts are true. They place all their expectations on us, leaving the child little room to explore their personality freely. Adult ideas can be overwhelming to children. These ideals may not be true but will become valid only when the child agrees. For example, my mom repeatedly told me I was a great dancer and, one day, a single person told me I could not dance and that I should stop embarrassing myself. At that moment, I thought everything my mom said was a lie and that I could not, in fact, dance at all.

After that, I stopped dancing altogether and never mentioned it again. However, that beat and passion inside of me never died. In 2010, I stumbled into a Zumba class at a Gold's Gym in North Carolina. I did not know what it was, but the class was packed, and the trainer up front told me I could burn up to 1000 calories in an hour. I fell in love with this dance fitness class so much that I started coming to the gym twice a day. I lost 25 lbs. in about three months, and I wasn't even trying to lose it. I was so passionate that instructors would often call me to the front to demonstrate the moves. But I was still stuck in that one person's belief. For years, I stayed great yet danced in the back where no one could see me. One day, someone else believed in me more than I did in myself. Then, I read self-help books and made personal development a part of my daily life. Finally, I took a terrifying leap of faith and became an instructor eight years after entering my first Zumba class. Imagine if I did not believe that one person's negative opinion? Maybe I would have been a backup dancer for Janet or Bey, and perhaps I would have attended the prestigious *Alvin Ailey Dance Company*; the world may never know. What are you in agreement with that is untrue? This guide will help you let go of those falsehoods, and you will grow into the woman you imagined yourself to be.

After graduating high school, I joined the military. I come from a military family; I was born near an army base; and, at the time, it seemed like the most logical thing to do. I was super excited though I did have to put my dreams of becoming the next *Cicely Tyson* on hold. In between being active, I loved to do stage plays. I would just come alive on stage. I got to pretend to be someone else for a while, which meant I did not have to be myself. But I could not sing or dance according to other people's (non-factors) opinions, I was dead broke, and I had no problem putting that "little dream" on hold. "Be all that you can be, in the Army," I would sing in my head. I was what they called gung-ho: *unthinkingly enthusiastic and eager, especially about taking part in fighting or warfare: "the gung-ho soldier who wants all the big military toys,"* according to Webster's Dictionary. I was so eager and excited that I overlooked the cost and consequences of injury.

I completed four years in the Army, and about halfway through my military career, I injured myself. Although my activity slowed down, my body had gotten used to burning energy at a high level. My body started to store the fat I was no longer burning so I started gaining weight, but it didn't bother me. I always wanted to gain weight. Over the next ten years, I would give birth to 2 kids, complete a marriage and divorce, and bury my parents. One day, I looked up and I had gained 80 lbs. *Woosaahh.* I had no idea until a friend of mine snapped a photo of me. Those little ounces crept up out of nowhere. I sent the picture back, like, "Harpo, who dis woman in my outfit?" "Um, fool, that is you!" WOW. That was a game-changer for me. I decided I must lose weight now, and I started eating rabbit food and starving myself. I didn't eat well, and I ended up malnourished. That did not work. I would lose weight and gain it back because I wasn't practicing sustainable techniques. I wanted quick microwave results, and we all know that food is cold and nasty in the middle.

No, thank you. On top of all that, I was devastated by my legs and back injury. It was almost like I couldn't be who I thought I was. I couldn't control my weight, health, or emotional eating. But I was a health coach; shouldn't I know how to do all this stuff? I felt like giving up on my goals, dissolving my company, and moving on to something else. But something in me was wrestling with the thought of giving up. I felt convicted in my spirit. Then, two amazing things happened. I started talking to God about my feelings. Nothing formal, just a quick, "Hey God, I'm not sure about this, throw me a sign if you think I should stay, thanks to Big Guy, Amen." I'm a simple girl and, often, I am short for words, but God heard my heart. I received an opportunity I could not refuse. Teaching classes in a beautiful event hall was always a dream. My first instinct was to turn it down. I didn't even respond for three days. I was truly going to say that I could not do it. But the Holy Spirit began to press upon me. It indeed was not about me or my feelings, so I grabbed the opportunity, unsure of what God was going to do next. Then, I got the complete download for this book. I was overwhelmed. "*I can't do that. No one is going to read it; I don't know where to start,*" I had every excuse known to humankind. "*Sis, stop making excuses,*" I heard loud and clear. I heard in my spirit that I would need a coach and an accountability partner. God truly knows you better than you know yourself. Trust Him and trust the process.

I have been researching information for this book over the last ten years. Only, I never had the confidence to write and put it all together. It is the book I wish I had on my journey. This guide will teach you how to reorient your thought process about food and how you eat it. The food industry has done a remarkable job in marketing by creating billboards, commercials, and displays; even the supermarket entrance right at the bakery. Even if you weren't thinking of a dessert, you are now. That is a setup for those of us with food addictions! My reward receptors start going "Bing, Bing, Bing, ting, ting, ting." We will discuss your reward receptors in detail later in the habit section of this book.

The book includes eight modules. The course is self-paced and will take 8-12 weeks to complete. In part one, we will break down the mind and how it is hindering or helping us through this process. Next, we get into finding your motivation and your "Why" for starting this process. We dedicated almost a whole week to this because it is the most significant factor in your ability to maintain your progress without giving up. We will cover the effects of putting your health on the "back burner." In weeks three and four, we begin creating new healthy habits. The tools to undo old habits and create new ones are included here. The idea is to get you to a place where the tools in this book become habits in your life. Like breathing, you don't think about breathing; you just do it. Upon completing the course, you will have lifetime access to our fitness community, all the tools and documents associated with the course, and any training video or workout videos created for The Slay Academy. The course is not a challenge; this is a lifestyle change. This manual will break down everything you need to know about nutrition and fitness. We also focus on healing, rest, and recovery; and we begin to apply all the tools to our daily lives. The last week of the course is all about maintenance and survival. We often talk about getting to the goal, but how do we stay at the top once we reach it? A fall from the top could be devastating. Therefore, we learn how to avoid this at all costs. The book is about what worked for me, the resources I used, and the lessons I learned so that you can avoid those typical mistakes. Once you complete this course, the real work begins. But you will have more than enough tools to be successful. Upon completion, you will understand how and why you have particular eating habits. You will learn how to analyze the thought process of the way you are eating.

Weight loss should be peaceful; understanding the foundation of your relationship with your food is critical in this process. Rather than teach you another diet plan, I decided to focus on a behavior modification course. Changing your relationship with food will be a slow process. However, the sacrifice should not be brutal. Let's face it; if it were easy, we would already have done it. The tools in this program can be adjusted to fit everyone's specific needs. The course can be a marathon and a sprint. Let the marathon continue and move with urgency as our lives depend on it. We will spend the next 8-12 weeks getting to know ourselves again.

Module 1 – Mindset Shift

"The body that you want already exists; we just have to find her, love her, heal her and hang on to her." – Slay Body

Learning Objectives:

- ✓ Participants will be able to set intentions for the course and life
- ✓ Participants will spend time setting their expectations for the course
- ✓ Understand the importance of Abundance Mindset

Coach's Corner: Coaches will teach participants how important it is to create a mind shift at the beginning of this journey. Participants must agree with the process and agree to finish the process. Most fitness and health experts say that the battle is 80% nutrition and 20% fitness. I say it's 100% mindset.

Time: 2 hours or two sessions

<u>Intro to Module 1:</u>

I am sure there are many reasons you chose to read this book. I needed a step-by-step guide for this process. I mean, even at my corporate job, I recently asked my manager for a step-by-step guide, and she looked at me like I was crazy - the nerve! She proceeded to hand me several books and guidelines to assist me with my daily work. I was grateful because it was a plethora of information. The only problem was that it was too much information, and it was extremely time-consuming to find what I needed.

At the start of this book, I am at the end of myself. I was over the up and down weight fluctuations, starting a challenge only to quit mid-way through, and receiving a not-so-good report from my healthcare provider. I was sick of myself. I had to get my heart right to move forward without being inundated with those negative thoughts telling me my goals were impossible. My Grandmother would always say, "Baby, you can do anything through Christ Jesus." As a kid, I thought it was just cliché, but this Bible verse got me off the couch, and I grabbed a pen and paper. I needed a plan and a little more Jesus.

Human beings tend to compare themselves to others constantly. We all want to fix what we can see, right? I know that if you picked up this book, we are fixers, like Olivia Pope. We see a problem; consider it handled! So, we get caught up in trying to fix that post-pregnancy pooch, love-handles, flabby arms; so much so that, if you are like me, you've considered or had surgery to rectify this situation because we are about solutions. Only temporarily fixing what we see is merely treating a symptom to a much bigger problem. And thanks to good old social media, we constantly see others' "good days" photoshopped pictures with great angles, oh and "Julie lost 40 pounds in 30 days, so what on earth is wrong with me?"

We think, 'I want to look that way,' and when it does not happen in 2 weeks, we give up or get the surgery. We will break down the appropriate timing for goal setting later in this book. For now, we must fix the inside first and foremost. The mind is a brilliant masterpiece. The mind is what controls every part of your life. I am not trying to be uber religious here, but literally, I had to pray to God for a paradigm mind shift to get my heart right. I tried this on my own with fleeting results. Meaning, I would start strong; as soon as I got busy or lazy, I would forget all about my goals! I wanted to mention this because it may help you as well. Folks told me how God helped them overcome their weight loss and health struggles for so many years. I thought I wouldn't bother God with such minor issues; losing weight is easy, I got this. After a few years of not getting it done or coming close and falling off, I finally reached out to God.

Here is my prayer for you: It will move mountains.

Dear Father,

Search me, oh God. Please help me find any discrepancies that may hinder my success in this process. Lord, I am stuck, and I need you. This issue has become a giant in my life. And like David, I came to slay this giant. Father, I thank you in advance for healing our bodies right now, Lord. I forgive myself for all the damage I may have caused. But God, you are a redeemer, and you promised me that I would have life and have it more abundantly. I pray for victory over cravings, late-night snacking, and stress eating. Lord bind up anything in our way, give us complete freedom in this area in our lives, and we come against any negative self-talk. Today, we break every chain holding us back from becoming who you said we were born to be. And I declare that you will give us healed hearts and whole, healthy bodies. The strategies found here will mend the broken heart. I pray for ease in understanding how food and exercise affects our overall health. Amen.

Insert your prayer request:

_____

_____

_____

_____

_____

_____

_____

_____

_____

_____

_____

_____.

Let's begin -

Action Step 1: Find your inner peace

o **Task 1: Reduce Negative Thoughts**

1. Negative thoughts are normal - Experts estimate that the mind thinks between 60,000 – 80,000 thoughts a day, and about 80% are negative. Ouch! There isn't a way to make these stop, unfortunately. However, we can control how we respond to them.

2. Prepare your day - a 5-minute meditation session each morning

Coach's Corner: Share a story with the participants. For example, my therapist used to say, "If you go to work on level 8, it is likely you will hit level 10 by the end of the day because we can't control what others do." However, if I work on a level 1 or 2, I may only reach level 4 by the end of the day. Hey, a 5-minute meditation session can alter your entire day and keep you from blowing up. And this further puts us at a deficit toward our goal. Stress releases cortisol, which produces stubborn fat, such as belly fat. A lose/lose situation.

Weight loss, healthy habits, and discipline are the highest forms of self-love. If you're not practicing self-discipline in all areas of your life, you are not adequately caring for the temple given to you to house your spirit. For example, I dread cleaning my house. However, someone must do it. About halfway through the chore, something clicks, and I start to feel outstanding and accomplished. At some point, I don't want to stop cleaning, and I will clean until the point of exhaustion. Crazy, huh? Not really. Seeing the house messy was causing me severe anxiety. I was constantly thinking about it, and I could not rest peacefully in a junky place. During that cleaning, I began to release pent-up energy and negative emotions.

Removing clutter from my environment created a cleaner, more comfortable atmosphere. I was able to feel happier and more relaxed. It turns out that clutter profoundly affects our mood and self-esteem. The self-discipline of tidying up is a form of self-care. When Mary J. Blige blasts through my crib, you know it's cleaning time. I even pencil in cleaning on my rest days from workouts. I hate missing workouts because it affects my mood, but if I get in a vigorous cleaning session, I can have a peaceful home and release endorphins simultaneously. Does this make sense? The things we dread the most can be forms of self-care. Find your peace. If that means losing weight so that your anxiety will not cause you to beat yourself up about your shortcomings continuously, you are in the right place.

Focus-Practice Manifestation (FPM) is the public display of emotion or feeling or bringing something theoretical to reality. Would you believe me if I told you I could manifest all your dreams into reality? You can manifest anything you want or desire into your life. Love, money, and your dreams can become real through the power of attraction and belief. Where energy goes, success flows. But first, know exactly what you want, and please be specific about it. You can also manifest negativity into your life. It is imperative to focus on what you want rather than what you **don't** want. We begin the course and end the course with this practice.

o **Task 2: Set Your Specific Intention**

1. Once you've set your particular intention, ask for what you want aloud and then write it. Write the vision and make it clear. And yes, that includes your goal weight. Have a vision for every part of your life.

_____

_____

_____

_____

_____

_____

o **Task 3: Visualization (In-Class)**

1. Take 5 minutes to visualize yourself as the woman you dream of being. See her living her best life in the dream you just manifested. What does she like to eat? What time does she wake up in the morning? What is her favorite color? Does she have a job or own a business? Visualize every detail about that woman because she is already inside you, waiting to emerge.

o **Task 4: Future You (Homework) – (Coach show example)**

1. Create a Future Box- Find a small box or shoebox and place any and everything in that box that represents your intention. You will begin to channel positive energy towards your intention, making the vision crystal clear. You can also write on sheets of paper and place them inside the box. Once we complete goal setting, you will determine the date to reopen your Future Box. In the meantime, decorate your box and have fun!

Write a letter to your future self - another excellent manifestation tool.

✓   Imagine talking to a friend. After all, your inner dream woman is about to become your best friend. The letter should be positive, uplifting, and full of gratitude. Thank her for showing up and supporting you through this process. You can hand write this letter and place it in your Future Box, or you can visit the website futureme.org. You can type your letter there and pick a date to deliver it to your email. I think this rocks. I like to write letters for my 1-year future self, 5-year future self, and 10-year future self, but you can pick any date. Just make sure you give yourself enough time and grace to change.

Action Step 2: Create a Personal Development Plan

Coach's Corner: Now that we have let the universe know what we want. Let's start taking steps to reach our dreams. Yes, we can manifest, but we must put in the work. All know, faith without works is dead, right? You cannot reach optimal success with a negative mindset. Personal development changed my life. It is a practice that I started about four years ago. You will need to add this practice to your life for continued growth permanently.

Personal development is a lifelong process. It is a way for people to assess their skills, set goals, and realize maximum potential. Personal development helped me in the area of choice. Choices are a massive part of this process. Every morning we have the power to make a better choice. If I hit my snooze button and I am subsequently late for work, that is my fault. I chose to hit the snooze button, so technically, I can't get mad at the traffic jam on my way to work.

This thought process freed me from living in offense all the time and removed a ton of stress from my life. Personal development will help you make relevant, positive, and practical life choices and process decisions for your future to enable personal empowerment. Maslow (1970) suggests that all individuals have an in-built need for personal development through self-actualization (Maslow's Hierarchy of Needs). Self-actualization refers to the desire that everybody has 'to become everything that they are capable of becoming.' In other words, it relates to self-fulfillment and the need to reach full potential as a unique human being. That explains it.

Our desire to reach our fullest potential will hang in the balance, and we will always feel unfilled with life until we realize our highest potential. Many people say that they have a great job but are unfulfilled. You have areas in your life that have not reached their highest growth. This feeling of incompleteness means that you have not fulfilled your purpose, have not reached your ultimate health goals, or have neglected essential mind and body self-care. When you continuously work on yourself, you are more likely to reach your full potential. When practicing PD, you should focus on any activity that improves self-awareness and identity, develops skills and growth, enhances life quality, and helps you bring your hopes and dreams to life.

o **Task 1: Integrate Physical Activity**
1. While conducting the physical activity, be prepared to include a form of encouragement. A self-help audiobook, a personal development video on YouTube, or some upbeat, positive music are great places to start. My favorite thing to do is get on the elliptical and blast *Tony Robbins* in my earbuds. When I get off the machine, I am usually a crying

ball of emotions because I just leveled up. You may have to turn social media, the news, and the TV off. Feed your mind with positivity constantly. Do this every single day and watch your results explode like magic.

o **Task 2: Journaling**

1. It is often a good idea to keep a journal of your personal development. Write down critical developments in your learning process. In 1 year, you want to reflect on your development journey. It is also a great idea to start a gratitude journal. Gratitude will help the mind shift from focusing on negative thoughts to positive ones.

2. Begin and end each day with reflection and gratitude.

o **Task 3: Affirmations**

Coach's Corner: Give Participants examples of goal-oriented affirmations.

- ✓ What weaknesses do we need to overcome?
- ✓ What struggles do you have? Be intentional.
- ✓ Set Intentions to your affirmations
- ✓ Remind yourself who you are
- ✓ Re-introduce yourself

o **Task 4: I Am Enough Activity**

Meditating is a tool to help you stay on track with your goals. Meditation simply means to engage in mental exercises such as concentrating on one's breathing or repetition of a mantra to reach a heightened level of spiritual awareness. This practice is all about understanding. I am not an expert on this, but I do practice it, and it has helped me tremendously. It helps me bring everything back into focus from being pulled in many directions. You can purchase meditation music, listen for free online, or just sit in silence. By the end of the day, we are exhausted and have little to give to our families. Meditation helps you get back to the bigger picture.

Coach's Corner: There are many different forms of meditation.
- ✓ (Example) Type into Google: *meditation for weight loss*, and you will see so many tools to assist you with this.
- ✓ Audiobooks also give you more assistance and a deeper understanding of this practice. Try it for at least 30 days before you throw in the towel on this one.

Let's give it a try now; it only takes 2 minutes.

☐ Breath in deeply for 4 seconds; hold your breath for 4 seconds and blow the breath out for 4 seconds. Repeat.
☐ Now close your eyes. Again, breathe in deeply for 4 seconds, hold the breath for 4 seconds, and blow the breath out for 4 seconds.

☐ Now hold the right nostril closed. Again, breathe in deeply 4 seconds, hold the breath for 4 seconds, and blow out for 4 seconds.

☐ Now hold the left nostril closed. Again breathe in deeply 4 seconds, hold the breath for 4 seconds, and blow out for 4 seconds.

Your body should feel relaxed and free, and some tension may even be relieved. Open your eyes, your vision should be more precise, and your body should be calmer. You just gave your body all the oxygen it needs to thrive. You can do this anywhere - at the office, in bed, sitting in a chair, or while driving through a traffic jam; just keep your eyes open for that last one.

Prayer – always talk freely, express gratitude, and present prayer requests. Prayer is another form of meditation. Only mindful meditation is usually silent unless you may be repeating a mantra.

As I mentioned before, prayer is a great tool to lead this journey. It's one of the easiest; you just talk to God; He is always available. Open up to God like you would to a best friend. Mindful meditation is what I like to use when I need to hear what God has to say.

Reading is also a form of meditation. What does the Bible say about weight loss? Bust open that Bible, honey; dig deeper and meditate on His word.

✓ *1 Corinthians 6:19-20 (NASB1995)*

"Or do you not know that your body is a temple of the Holy Spirit who is in you, whom you have from God, and that you are not your own? For you have been bought with a price: therefore glorify God in your body."

✓ *1 Corinthians 10:13 (NASB)*

"No temptation has overtaken you except *something* common to mankind; and God is faithful, so He will not allow you be tempted beyond what you are able, but with the temptation will provide the way of escape also, so that you will be able to endure it."

✓ *Romans 12:1 (NASB)*

"Therefore I urge you, brothers *and sisters*, by the mercies of God, to present your bodies as a living and holy sacrifice, acceptable to God, *which is* your spiritual worship."

✓ *1 Corinthians 10:31 (NIV)*

"So whether you eat or drink or whatever you do, do it all for the glory of God."

✓ *Galatians 5:22-23 (NASB)*

"But the fruit of the Spirit is love, joy, peace, patience, kindness, goodness, faithfulness, gentleness, self-control; against such things, there is no law."

✓ *Proverbs 25:27 (NIV)*

"It is not good to eat too much honey, nor is it honorable to search out matters that are too deep."

✓ *Ephesians 2:10 (NIV)*

"For we are God's handiwork, created in Christ Jesus to do good works, which God prepared in advance for us to do."

✓ *Galatians 1:10 (NIV)*

"Am I now trying to win the approval of human beings or of God? Or am I trying to please people? If I were still trying to please people, I would not be a servant of Christ."

✓ *James 4:17 (NIV)*

"If anyone, then, knows the good they ought to do and doesn't do it, it is a sin for them."

- ➢ Write the Scriptures on notecards, add reminders to your phone
- ➢ Use a dry-erase marker to write the Bible verses on your bathroom mirror
- ➢ Make the verse the lock screen on your phone
- ➢ Purchase a daily devotional (*visit* The Slay Academy | Slay Body Fitness www.slaybodyfitness.com/theslayacademy *for recommendations*)
- ➢ Use the verses to combat negative self-talk
- ➢ Check out https://soveryblessed.com/10-bible-verses-for-your-weight-loss-journey/https://soveryblessed.com/10-bible-verses-for-your-weight-loss-journey/ . And download the Bible verse for the weight loss card.

o **Task 5: Identify If You Are in Emotional Turmoil**

✓ Exhausted all the time/ low energy

✓ Distracted

✓ Inability to focus

✓ Avoidance

✓ Angry/Moody

(Practice the exercises above to help you get centered and overcome this turmoil before moving forward).

Activity/Homework

Practice being intentional in everything that you do.
Give 100% to every duty that you are privileged to complete.
Instead of saying, "I must do this", practice saying, "I *get* to do this."

✓ Begin the practice of journaling for 5 minutes each morning and each night. Practice Gratitude.

✓ Each week add a new mental strength activity to your daily planner (see The Slay Academy | Slay Body Fitness www.slaybodyfitness.com/theslayacademy)

✓ Future Box

✓ Future Me Letter

✓ Repeat affirmations each morning for 60 seconds. Write them down on a piece of paper or the bathroom mirror with a dry erase marker and say them over and over for 1 minute. (Sample included in appendix)

Module 2 – Superpower

Those who have a 'why' to live can bear almost any 'how.'" – *Viktor Frankl.*

Learning Objectives:
- ✓ Participants will be able to determine their *Why.*
- ✓ Participants will be able to create a Mantra.
- ✓ Participants will explain why motivation is a crucial factor.
- ✓ Each participant will be assigned journal entries and will leave the session understanding how to track energy and journal daily.
- ✓ Participants will identify mental distractions and dig deep to find what holds them back from their dream life.

Time: 90 Minutes

Coaches Corner: Your WHY is your superpower! This journey can be the best ride of your life some days. And, other days, it is an all-out war. Your reason for embarking on this journey is the most critical step at the beginning and throughout. Will power, simply put, is not enough. As humans, we often have an influx of emotions and hormones out of our control. So, you guessed it right, that chocolate cake would not stand a chance on any day of the PMS cycle. For most of us, the urge to eat junk and the loss of willpower is insane during this time of the month. However, my WHY is to be here for my children and provide a long-lasting legacy for my family. So, when I compare that "WHY" to chocolate cake - "Bye, Felicia," I wave to the cake. Winning!

Intro to Module 2

In this section of the course, we will take a deep dive into your life to help you discover your WHY. This is a life transformation; therefore, it could take several months or years to reach your ultimate life goal. I know this because I am on this journey continuously. What is going to get you up and motivated day after day? You will be exhausted, especially moments before your breakthrough. Your WHY is the foundation of your passion and the fuel to ignite your persistence. How to lose weight is irrelevant without your superpower. You will need something other than willpower to hold you up, so that you don't fall back into old behaviors. To be successful on this journey, you must prepare to put in more effort. But not necessarily physical work. The work includes planning and organizing until your new healthy lifestyle is on autopilot. Your desire and motivation are critical to your success. Relying on your superpower allows you to grow through the rough patches and stop the pitfall of New Year's resolution let downs and the good old, "I will start as soon as…", but 'as soon as' never comes.

Here is a great example to understand how powerful your why can be. When my son was two years old, he ran out into traffic. I immediately jumped over a parked car and launched for my son like I was Superwoman without question or thought. If someone paid me to jump over that car, I would not and probably could not do it. No way! But my WHY (my son) was in life-or-death danger, and nothing would have stopped me from jumping. As you can see, you cannot just choose to do this. You must activate your superpower because life will happen.

Tell yourself, "I get to do this," rather than, "I have to do this," or "I hate going to the gym." The truth is we are very motivated to be lazy and accomplish tasks with the least effort possible. The principle of most minor action, energy, or resistance is very common. What's the fastest way to get to the next destination? A straight line, right? That is great for most activities, but we streamline the process to get the most out of each workout and meal in fitness. It may not always be a straight line; modifications and variations help enhance this journey. Go ahead and stop beating yourself up for feeling lazy; it's natural. In this course, we will use our WHY to overcome this feeling of laziness or least effort. Without your WHY, your goals will become futile, meaning it is merely a want rather than a need.

Let's begin –

Action Step 1: Find your WHY

o **Task 1: Complete Questionnaire**

1. Why do you want to lose weight?
2. Why is it important to you?
3. Do you have any health concerns? Family history?
4. What gets you out of bed in the morning?
5. What circumstances give you feelings of hope?
6. When you've reached goals in the past, what was the reason?
7. Who do you know and look up to that has shared their 'why'?
8. Who in the health and fitness world do you admire?
9. What does a day look like if you live your healthiest life?
10. What would be different in your life if you achieved your health or weight loss goals?
11. What do you want people to think about you?
12. What do you want to think about yourself?
13. What do you imagine happening when you reach your goals?
14. How do you want people to remember you when you die?
15. What activities consume your thoughts and make you forget about your problems and life?
16. What are you holding back? Is there more?
17. What are your core values?

o **Task 2: Write Down Your WHY**

1. Write down your WHY and post it somewhere you can see it daily.

2. Keep a journal

• Write down your thoughts on good days and hard days. Record the things that help you power through your good days. What hindered you or caused the bad days? Recording your daily events will help you identify patterns and habits. More challenging days require more motivation and an increasing need to lean on your WHY.

o **Task 3: Visualize Your Why**

1. Surround yourself with photos of your WHY

2. Picture your WHY when things get challenging

o **Task 4: Remember to Renew Your WHY.**

1. Revisit the questionnaire every 90 days to see if you can add your why.

o **Task 5: Talk to a Friend or Therapist**

1. Am I sabotaging my weight loss?

2. Is procrastination a factor in my life?

3. Dig deeper!

4. Are you sleepwalking through your life?

5. Do you have a reason to live?

6. Understand achievement vs. fulfillment?

Action Step 2: Find Your Power Hour

• The Power Hour can be a significant motivating factor. It is the period you are most productive. I call it primetime. My primetime or Power Hours are between 6 am and 10 am. This time of the day gets the bulk of my energy. I schedule my most important activities during this time. I prefer to work out during this time because I know I will give maximum effort. My attitude is much better. My nightly workouts are full of whining and complaining because I'm tired, and those are not my power hours. Learning this about yourself will help you overcome your feelings of guilt and unworthiness.

o **Task 1: Discover When You Are Most in the Zone**
1. Visualization exercise - when do you feel most energized
2. Download the slay fit energy tracker- monitor your energy levels for 2-3 days
3. Block out the hours when you're at your peak, when you have moderate amounts of energy, and when you typically feel sluggish, and color code them on your daily calendar.

o **Task 2: When Do You Zone Out?**
1. Visualize times when you easily zone out. What time of day is it?
2. Concentrate on low focus tasks during these times
3. Focus on low level exercises, i.e. walking outside

Action Step 3: Create Your Mantra

My Mantra: I will work just as hard on myself as I do for others. I want to feel good in my body, and I want to create the best version of myself to help and encourage others. It is essential to be here for my future grandkids.

o **Task 1: What Do You Want?**

1. Write down what you desire most, at this moment, right now.

o **Task 2: Declarative Statements**

1. Turn what you desire into a declarative statement. Use first person. Avoid negative words (not, never, won't, etc.).

o **Task 3: Write, Cite, Repeat.**

1. Be sure it is authentic to you versus meeting the approval or reviews of your peers. Test your words by writing, citing, and repeating them, especially in crucial moments that will challenge you.

Action Step 4: Rip Up Your Laziness Contract!

o **Task 1: Make a Commitment to Yourself**

Get out a piece of blank paper and write the following:

1. **I abandon the thought that I am just lazy**
2. **I abandon the agreement I made as a child that I was lazy**

3. **I abandon the agreement I made with others when they called me lazy**
4. **I abandon the thought that this journey is too hard**
5. **I abandon the thought that I am not good enough**

➤ Feel free to add more

o **Task 2: Now, Rip Up the Contract!**

1. Rip it up or shred it.
2. Burn this if you have a safe place like the fireplace.
3. I hereby release you from all negative agreements!

Action Step 5: Do Not Accept Anything Below Your Goals!

o **Task 1: Never Settle!**

1. Your dream is worth fighting for
2. You are not average!

o **Task 2: Visualize What Is on the Other Side**

Module 3 – Goal setting
"Your Business Plan for Life"

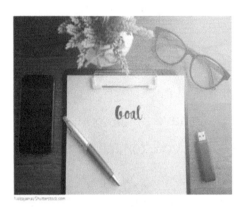

Learning Objectives:

✓ Create bite-sized goals to help let go of doubt.

✓ Understand the meaning of SMART goals

✓ Understand delayed gratification and how it affects goals.

✓ Insert goals into goal tracking applications.

✓ Apply milestones to long-term goals.

✓ Create short-term vs. long-term goals.

Time: 2 hours or two sessions

Intro to Module 3:

Ask yourself, "What do I want in life?" Now, imagine that everything you want already exists. Next, ask yourself, "Who do I need to become to create the lifestyle of my dreams?" It was a life-changing process for me. I looked up to many successful women in my life. I used to think, 'Man, I wish I could be like her.' I would soon learn the reasons why I admired these women. It was because the attributes and core values these women possessed were already inside of me. At that moment of realization, I decided to become the woman of my dreams. She would show up in my dreams, and I would daydream about her all the time. I even made-up fictional stories about her.

I asked myself, 'What qualities and attributes does she have? How can I obtain this magic?' I identified the character, behaviors, and attitude I needed to become my dream person. I started becoming a new being, and doors began to swing open in the areas of love, relationships, finance, spirituality, and overall health. I was becoming her, the lady of my dreams. Start dreaming about the possibilities of your future. How many hours would you like to work or not work? Do you want to own a business or grow your business? How do you want to feel when you wake up in the morning? Your goals will provide clear and specific direction; you can become whoever you want to be. Find the direction you want to go in and begin to build consistent habits to get you there. At her fullest potential, my dream lady is working her business full-time, feeling good in her body, and not tethered to prescriptions. She is healthy in her old age so that her children will not have to care for her around the clock. She is a mentor, a coach, a philanthropist, a mom, a friend, a wife, a sister, and travels the world uplifting the masses, serving God in her ministry. Sis is All That! By imagining your dream life, you are activating the laws of attraction. Always dream bigger. My friend in my head, Joyce Meyer, told us, "You will never exceed your highest expectation."

What are you expecting from this journey? Write it down, and always show up with the highest expectation ready to receive. Write another letter to your future self. (See futureme.com) Explain your expectations. What is your hope? At the end of the 8-week course, review the letter to see if it aligns with your expectations. Where energy goes, focus flows. We need to get our minds to come in agreement with our goals or they simply will not work. In goal setting, it is uber important to write each goal down. Successful people know what they want and how they plan to get there. You cannot do this haphazardly. Without a clear, written plan, you will look up a year from now and be in the same spot you are in right now. Now, we will focus on your specific goals. Every part of your life matters in this transformation series, and we will set goals for all areas in life as we focus on whole health. These could be business goals and milestones, financial goals, and overall whole, healthy lifestyle goals. What habits and behaviors do you need to eliminate, and which behaviors do you need to reinforce? Let's get into it.

Action Step 1: Discover Who You Want to Become

o **Task 1: Entertainment versus Development**

1. Track your entertainment versus personal development ratio

2. Track all items you do each month consistently. Then compare the entertainment factor versus the personal development factor.

3. See the below examples.

• For more help, see the PDF Entertainment ratio tracker at The Slay Academy | Slay Body Fitness www.slaybodyfitness.com/theslayacademy

> ➢ How much tv do you watch daily? _____ (be as accurate as possible)
> ➢ How much time do you spend on social media?
> ➢ How much time do you spend learning a new skill?
> ➢ How much time do you spend reading books?

Action step 2: Write Down Your Goal (plant the seed)

o **Task 1: Start with small goals**

i.e. I want to lose 5 lbs. in 30 days.

• This goal is attainable and will help you stay committed without feeling like a failure. Setting goals too big often leads to sabotage. I set this goal for myself and lost 10 lbs. that month. The feeling of euphoria filled my desire to keep going. We will work on bigger goals later in this course.

o **Task 2: Evaluate the goal**

1. Is a goal weight realistic? A weight goal can be a great metric to track; however, do not be tied to one metric. Understanding that the scale will go up and down during this process is key to your success. I gave up so many times due to the variations of the scale. I thought this wasn't for me, and I must have been doing it all wrong. The truth is this new lifestyle will introduce new habits, foods, and surroundings. It will act accordingly, and each person's response will vary throughout the month. Do not be discouraged by the ebbs and flows of the scale. The best metric is 1- 2 pounds per week. Some months you may lose 15 lbs. and, during other months, the scale won't budge or may even go up. However, the average between each month of work should be 4-8 pounds. Remember, you are not just a number on a scale.

2. Is this Goal SMART?

□ S- Specific: The goal should be exact with no room for misinterpretation.

☐ M- Measurable/Meaningful: The goal should be quantifiable and the progress easy to track.

☐ A- Achievable: The goal should be attainable — not outlandish or unrealistic.

☐ R- Realistic: The goal should contribute to your broader, overarching goals.

☐ T- Time-sensitive: The goal should have a defined start and end date.

- "I want to lose 10 lbs. in the next three weeks using the slay academy method."

- SMART *Goal Reference Chart*

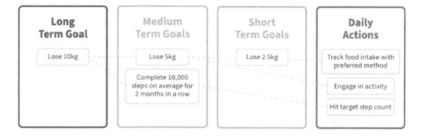

✓ Specific: I will start a drop shipping business.
✓ Measurable: I will work on my business for 1 hour each day, and the goal is to land my first sale within two weeks.

✓ Achievable: I have watched some videos on drop shipping and know that I can use Shopify and Oberto to start a business quickly.

✓ Relevant: I want to quit my job, work from home, and be my boss.

✓ Time-bound: I will begin on Saturday and land my first sale within two weeks.

Make your goal doable. Can you change your goal from 2 months to 2 years? Careful not to make the goal too small or too short. A small goal doesn't always mean short time frames. For instance, instead of saying, "I want to lose 20 lbs. in 2 months," say, "I want to lose 20lbs in 1 year." Just saying that made me feel good about it. Making our goals too short puts entirely too much pressure on our minds and body. Do not let any social media posts trick you; you want sustainable weight loss. However, I have too much experience, and I know these methods do not sustain a lifestyle change.

o **Task 3: List the Bad Habits**

1. Write what is hindering you from following your dreams

2. Identify triggers. i.e. I overeat while mindlessly eating or watching TV.

3. Find replacement options for events that trigger bad habits.

o **Task 4: List What Habits to Add**

Coach's Corner: Examples - clean out your pantry, so you aren't triggered by seeing snacks. Clean out your snack drawer. Avoid stress and anything that steals your joy. Eliminate it immediately. As we get to the end of our lives, we don't want to look back and say, "I spent too many years being aggravated and unhappy. I sacrificed all my health for what?" The opportunity cost is just too high.

o **Task 5: Replace Bad with Good**

1. Begin to think about replacing bad habits with good habits i.e. I will have water with my dinner rather than soda

o **Task 6: Download the 90-day Slay Fit Plan**

The 90-day plan is designed to help you reach optimal levels of success in your life. That plan breaks down everything taught throughout the modules and shows you how to implement them in your daily activities. Every 90 days, you will meet with your coach over the next 12 months, so that is four times per year. At the end of each 90 days, new habits will begin to develop, and you will see supernatural transformations across all sectors of your life.

> ➢ Fill this out at home and submit it for review at www.slaybodyfitness.com
> ➢ Schedule your first 90-day 1-on-1 consultation

o Task 7: Download Your Favorite Productivity Tracker app

Pro Tip: Only tracked goals will be achieved!

Action Step 2: Describe How you will delay gratification.

Coach's Corner: We are going to have to delay some things. The great thing is, we are delaying, not eliminating. For example, thirty days before Thanksgiving, I cut myself off from dessert until Thanksgiving Day. That way I can enjoy the holiday with family and friends without feeling guilty. Next, I get right back to my plan. No, I am not perfect. But 80 percent of your diet will carry you through the transformation. I am diligent in my eating habits for 5-6 days straight. Then I allow myself to relax just a little. This way, I never feel deprived, hungry, or suffering from lack.

Pro Tip: Gratification - the act of resisting an impulse to take an immediately available reward in the hope of obtaining a more-valued reward in the future. Your future goals are way more valuable. That cheesecake will be gone in a few minutes, and you may be stuck with the side effects of it forever. Everything is best in moderation.

o Task 1: List Things You Will Delay for Your Gratification

i.e. I will enjoy cake only at parties.

Action Step 3: Create Long-term Goals

• Long-term goals may take significant time or effort to achieve. A short-term goal typically takes less than a year to complete, while a long-term goal represents an achievement that could take a year or more. If you understand how to develop goals effectively, it can help you monitor your progress by adding milestones along the way.

o **Task 1: Use the Reference Table to Write Your Long-term Goals**

o **Task 2: Use Visualization Techniques**
1. Create a mental picture of what you want your life to look like at a specific point, such as five or ten years from now.

o **Task 3: Identify Challenges**
1. While setting your goals, take time to identify any obstacles you may encounter on your journey to achieving them. Don't wait until the war starts in order to put your armor on; show up ready to fight!

Action Step 4: Applying Milestones to Long-term Goals.

o **Task 1: Use Visualization Techniques**
1. Create a mental picture of what you want your life to look like at a specific point, such as five or ten years from now.

o **Task 2: Identify Challenges**

1. While setting your goals, take time to identify any obstacles you may encounter on your journey to achieving them.

Action Step 5: Homework

➤ Submit 90-day Slay Fit plan to instructor for review and feedback.

➤ Apply goal setting to your other areas of life

Module 4 - Nutrition the Slay Way! The Slay Academy Method

Disclaimer- consult your doctor or a licensed nutritionist (highly recommended) before changing your nutrition plan, especially if on medication.

"A true act of self-love is learning to love yourself by loving your body, just as it is." – Coach Mo.

Learning Objectives:

✓ Describe the 'Add-In" method

✓ Explain the 'Swap-method" method

✓ Complete a sample meal plan

✓ Create Meal prep cheat sheets

✓ Understand sustainable weight loss

✓ The Slay Academy Method (SAM)

✓ Understand the caloric deficit

Time: 3 hours or two weeks

Coach's Corner: Slay your nutrition; module 4 focuses on food with a twist. Participants will learn an approach to eating healthily and enjoyably. The Slay Academy Method (SAM) changes how we think and behave around food. It is not necessarily about knowing what to eat but rather how to eat. Also, how to control our emotions around food. Food and feelings often go hand in hand. Understanding what our emotions genuinely need can be the difference between success and failure. Also, we take a deep dive into what our body needs. The body has a language of its own. Using the tools learned in Module 1, participants should be strong in the walk with meditation and prayer. Meditation tools are great for learning to listen to the body and understand what it tells us.

We often treat or mistreat our bodies based on the amount of love and value we have for our bodies. If we hate our bodies, we will mistreat them. Therefore, we teach and encourage participants by lifting them to a higher vibration and giving them the tools to reach success beyond their limitations. Often, holding the pupil's hand for too long will enable them. Teach participants "how to fish" so they may eat and feed their generations properly, forever.

Intro to Module 4:

Help! I don't know what to eat. It is simply not about eating perfectly, but how to make nutrition empower your life rather than cause you guilt and frustration. Are you eating for comfort? We call these comfort foods because they make us feel suitable for the moment. The problem is, it numbs us temporarily; in the end, we will owe a considerable debt for the comfort we chose. It is not about being lazy; your mind has built habits and routines sabotaging your goals. What is the root of your suffering? Find the answer to this, and you find the power to control your behaviors.

This Module can be one of the most challenging modules in this course. However, this module will provide you with a step-by-step guide to slay your nutrition. Week 4 is a great week introducing SAM Nutrition- the slay way. Weight gain is a symptom. SAM is our method created to identify the cause and eradicate it. It is essential to do all the work in its entirety as your root cause could be different. All the work is necessary for this journey regardless of the root cause. It is proven that we get healthy to lose weight, not the other way around.

Focusing on weight loss can lead to yo-yo dieting, poor health outcomes, and wasted time. When this happens, one could get frustrated and quit the process altogether. Our number one goal of SAM is health over all other matters. The good news is weight loss is a side-effect of getting healthy. If weight loss were simply about a nutrition plan, it would not be so challenging for so many people. This course section will learn new eating habits, set healthy goals, and take our lives back from food. In module 1, we learned how to create healthy habits and implement them into our lives. Over the past several weeks, you have been challenged to develop and set goals effectively using habit tracking tools, meditation, and journaling. I am looking forward to implementing those tools again to help put your nutrition on autopilot, but you are the driver of your life. We will also break down emotional eating and why it is detrimental to healthy living. Emotional eating caused me so much grief. Let's focus on tools to help modify this behavior and build the life of your dreams.

Changing the "way" you eat has little to do with what you eat. Sustainable weight loss is obtained by giving your body the time to adjust to all the changes you are throwing at it. If you cause your body to lose 20 pounds in a week, it may eventually retaliate, and you could end up hurting the body more than helping it. Besides, healthy living has less to do with a number on a scale. Also, be mindful that results may be slow at first. But when the snowball effect occurs, things will get moving quickly and safely. It is like planting a seed. It seems to take forever at first, then next thing you know, there is a whole garden.

The SAM is also designed to decrease boredom and frustration at mealtime while avoiding extremes and time-consuming meal preps. Preparation is critical. However, we just don't want to spend too much time there, or we will not be able to sustain it with our already "full plates!" In this program, we avoid extremes as they cause too much stress, and mindset development will be a much more significant factor in successfully navigating the challenge of overwhelming goals and ideals. Finally, Module 4 provides an understanding of weight loss phases and an in-depth understanding of your current phase. Navigating the phases of your healthy journey is not about perfection but rather about character, discipline development, and consistency.

Let's assess the phases of your journey:

1. What 3 things are affecting your Health now?

_____, _____, _____

i.e., high blood pressure, shortness of breath)

2. Would removing any of these things change your life?

_____

3. What about your life feels unbalanced?

_____

Biologically? _____

Physiologically? _____

4. What can you do to achieve balance?

_____

5. What 3 things frustrate you about your body?

_____

_____

_____

6. How would removing one of these things make you feel?

_____

_____

_____

Action Step 1: Create a Healthy Relationship with Food/Fuel.

1. Ask these questions every time you feel like giving up:
   - Why am I suffering?
   - How am I handling stress?
   - Why do I keep quitting?

Many of us find ourselves in a situation-ship with our food! This 1st action step is vital for building a long-term healthy relationship with food. Below you will find several tasks to help end the food saga forever. Situation-ships are confusing to define and open to interpretation. The universal definition of a situation-ship is an undefined romantic relationship. And obviously, this is not a long-term relationship. Situation-ships may involve sex and romance, but they don't have the trajectory to move forward to a mature, loving relationship. Think of it essentially as short-term dating without a plan.

Situation-ships don't have any goals, terms, or purpose. Situation-ships are formed in the first place because of uncertainty. This peculiarity is simply unhealthy romantic relationships and food relationships. I used to tell myself that my bad habits were just temporary and that I would get my life together soon. This action led to situation-ship after situation-ship with food, leading to a downward spiral. Weight gain was the least of my worries. Slap on diabetes, cysts, constipation, fibroids, fibroadenomas, Hypertension, countless allergies, and poor gut health. If we can stop letting our emotions control us, we will make better decisions regarding food choices and ultimately have the life of our dreams.

We must understand that food is not a cure for emotions. If we can get down to the root cause and fix that, we can control our impulses when it comes to food habits. Food simply won't fix your problem; it adds a deeper layer of toxicity. If you want to get healthy, you must like yourself first. If you don't like yourself, your relationship with food will be a catastrophe.

o **Task 1: Implement Mindful Eating**

- Become present with what you are eating
- Eat at the table with no cell phone or tv
- Be aware of your feelings
- Do not eat at the computer
- Be mindful about your choices
- Plan your mealtime

o **Task 2: Identify the root cause of your emotional eating (Homework)**

Coach's Corner:
- ✓ *Go over the questions with the class*
- ✓ *Give examples*
- ✓ *Ensure class understanding*

> Assess your mood at each of the next seven meals by answering the questions below.

Pre-meal Questions:

1. Have you been present with your mind, body, and soul today?

(Explain to students that being present keeps them in tune with vision and goals and less likely to make poor decisions.)

2. Have you been stressed today?

Understand that stress eating will cause more frustration

3. What can you do to invite peace into your day?

Be aware and bring yourself back

4. Has negative self-talk invaded your space today?

5. Is the food fueling your goals or taking away from them?

6. Are you stressing about mealtime? Why?

7. What do you have to lose if you don't reach your goal?

After meal

1. How did the food make you feel?

2. Did you feel rushed?

3. Were you distracted?

4. Did you begin eating with a mindset of, 'I must eat all my food'?

5. Did the meal align with your why? Why or why not?

Assess these questions over the next week and write the answers in your journal. Do not obsess over every little detail but be patient with yourself. This time is about learning by yourself to strengthen your eating habits over time. If you had a cheat meal or dessert outside of reward day, it is essential to write it down and assess what happened, and not to beat yourself up about it—consistency over perfection. I guarantee you have ideally eaten over 80 percent of the time. Kudos to you!

o **Task 3: Listen to Your Body**
• What is your body telling you it needs? Stop and think.
• Are you truly hungry or bored?
• Are you dehydrated?
• Are you tired or sleepy?
• Are you upset or put off?
• Understand your body's language
• Assess yourself during the meal?
• Are you full halfway through?- your body is communicating with you
• Delayed gratification

Action Step 2: Create the Plate – The add-in/swap out Method

Pro Tip: The less restriction you place on your mind about eating, the less stress you will create around food. You will focus on the abundance of powerful foods to fuel the body. No single food or meal will determine how much weight you gain or lose. The less you restrict yourself completely, the less guilt you have about eating. (Share a story with a class about restrictions). The SAM formula focuses on the abundance of nourishment that you may indulge in rather than what you can't have. There are only a few restrictions on this plan.

The first one is to avoid any kind of soda, including diet soda. Here is why:

✓ Diet and regular sodas have both been linked to **obesity, kidney damage, and certain cancers**. Standard soft drinks have been related to elevated blood pressure.

✓ **Weight gain:** The high sugar content makes it one of the worst beverages you can drink. Drinking soda is a contributor to obesity in the United States.

✓ **Damages the teeth:** The various acids in soda cause tooth erosion. Also, the teeth play a significant role in digestion. We need healthy gums and teeth to be whole and healthy.

✓ **Increases Cancer Risk**: Certain types of soda, such as cola, contain caramel coloring. Avoid this as much as possible. Caramel coloring is made with ammonium compounds.

✓ **Accelerates Bone Loss:** The phosphate acid in soda is thought to interfere with calcium absorption, leading to a loss of bone mineral density.

✓ **Risk of Fatty Liver Disease:** Soda is often sweetened with high-fructose corn syrup with several negative health consequences, including non-alcoholic fatty liver disease.

Keep in mind that High Fructose corn syrup is banned in many countries.

✓ **Dangers of Artificial Sweeteners:** Most types of diet soda contain some kind of artificial sweetener. Sweeteners, such as sucralose (Splenda), saccharin, and aspartame, are associated with several health problems, including lupus, glucose intolerance, and multiple sclerosis. Aspartame, NutraSweet, and Equal are associated with increased brain tumors, mood disorders, declining mental function, migraines, and seizures.

✓ **Increased Risk of Diabetes:** Drinking soda also increases your risk of developing type 2 diabetes.

✓ **Benzene:** Benzene is a possible cancer-causing substance found in trim levels in some types of soda. It has been linked to Leukemia.

✓ **Increased the Risk of Rheumatoid Arthritis:** Drinking sugary soda may increase a woman's risk of developing rheumatoid arthritis

Reference:

www.webmd.com/diet/features/sodas-and-your-health-risks-debated

I hate restrictions; however, this is one that I implemented due to my sugar and soda addiction. The 2nd one is fried foods. This is just a temporary restriction and can be enjoyed on your day of indulgence.

o **Task 1: Calculate TDEE**

(This done with every 20 lbs. of weight loss)

TDEE stands for total daily energy expenditure. It is the total energy that a person uses in a day. TDEE is hard to measure accurately and varies day by day. More often, it is estimated using factors such as a person's basal metabolic rate (BMR), activity level, and the thermic effect of food.

BMR is a person's energy usage rate while resting in a temperate environment when the digestive system is inactive. In other words, it is the minimum energy needed to maintain a person's vital organs only. This calculator can be used to estimate your Total Daily Energy Expenditure (TDEE)
TDEE Calculator www.calculator.net/tdee-calculator.html

o **Task 2: Understand THE ELEMENTS**

Slay Academy Method Diet focuses on daily allowances, calorie deficit, and the perfect plate. The goal is to eat as many whole foods as possible at each meal. Snacks are allowed, but only after you have completed the daily allowance. Eventually, you begin to reach for your whole foods first. I often forget about the snack I was craving because my flesh was craving that snack, not my body. The goal is to create new habits.

The perfect PLATE has the following four elements

Keep It Simple Sis (KISS)

1. Vegetables

2. Protein- must be included in every meal.

Recommendation: 1 gram per pound of fat up to 250g

o Metabolism

o Hunger suppression

o Improved aging

o Lean muscle

o Healthy hair, skin, and nails

3. Carbohydrates- energy source, Curb hunger

4 Healthy Fats- Healthy fats support weight loss

Pro Tip: Your plate should **always** have these four elements

*See www.slaybodyfitness.com/theslayacademy for
shopping list

*See www.slaybodyfitness.com/theslayacademy for list of
foods

o **Task 3**: **Focus on these elements at each meal rather than the number of meals.**

o **Task 4**: **Snacking**

• 100 calories or less

• Don't plan to snack, but be prepared

• Snack only when necessary

o **Task 5: Swapping Out Method**

• Swap out your most challenging meal for a protein smoothie - do this 1x per day

• Swap out for healthier choices whenever possible

• Swap out fast food for home cooking

• Swap out processed snacks for home-baked goods

o **Task 6: Add-in Method**

• Add in more food if you are hungry

• If you crave candy, add in an apple. Eat the apple first.

• Add in foods that feel good to the body and eat them often

o Foods that make you feel alert

o Foods that make you feel energized

Action Step 3: Create Auto Slay

o **Task 1: Create a visual food diary**

o **Task 2: Before pics**

1. Post to the refrigerator or put it on your desk - not for everyone's view, though. This is between you and you.

o **Task 3: Redo your pantry**

o **Task 4: Set your eating schedule (Homework) –**

It does not matter how you split your calories up during the day. Do what feels natural to your body but try not to skip meals.

> ➤ Choose what works for YOU

> ➤ Choose how many meals you would like to eat

<u>Next four days:</u>

Day 1 (3 x meals)

Day 2 (5-6 small meals)

Day 3 (3 x meals)

Day 4 (5-6 small meals)

1. Do a self-assessment at the end of the four days

 ✓ Adjust based on your needs and feelings

Most days, I am well with two meals and a snack; however, some days, I need three meals. Don't be afraid to adjust if you make additional meals small; you will stay in the calorie deficit.

 ✓ If using the perfect plate - no need to count calories. But this is a good practice to use the first six weeks (see below). Understanding how to track my food was a game-changer. The perfect plate - Healthy Food Guide www.healthy

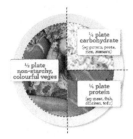

food.com/advice/the-perfect-plate/

Pro tip: the most important factor is being in a calorie deficit, no matter how many times you eat.

2. Download My Fitness Pal - Calorie tracker

✓ Food diary

✓ Food recall for three days of the week

✓ Photos of meals

✓ Calorie tracking

✓ Calorie + macro tracking

✓ Self-rating of dietary adherence

3. Common Habits and choices, but not required

✓ Eat Every 2 hours

✓ Fasting

✓ Track Calories

✓ Carb restriction

Action Step 4: Meet Your Battle Buddy (BB)- "Best Friend."

This journey will face many battles along the way. The best way to get through such storms is with a battle buddy. A battle buddy is a partner assigned to a soldier in the United States Army. Each battle buddy is expected to assist their partner in and out of combat. A Battle Buddy can save their fellow soldier's life by noticing negative thoughts and feelings and intervening to provide help. There is so much power in that. I knew that someone was assigned to me in the middle of a fight and would not leave me alone, no matter what. Some days, you will just need to know you are not alone in this fight.

o **Task 1: View Your Assigned Partner**

o **Task 2**: **Download Telegram**

o **Task 3: Reach Out to Your Partner and Introduce Yourself**

o **Task 4: Recite the Battle Buddy Creed**

This is my battle buddy. We are battle slayers. We did not come to play. We will check in weekly. We will send words of affirmation. I will encourage, remind, uplift. We will share tips, recipes, fitness hacks, successes, and failures. I will seek help from my BB when I am in despair.

Action Step 5: Set Small Achievable Goals.

o **Task 1: Keep It Simple Sis (KISS)**

o **Task 2: Work on controlling one meal at a time**

Action Step 6: Drink Your Weight Away!

o **Task 1: Eat Your Water**

Coach's Corner:

Teach participants and demonstrate which fruits and veggies will assist in water consumption

o **Task 2: Drink Half Your Body Weight in Ounces Daily**

Fluid weight gain is temporary; the more water you drink, the faster this weight is lost daily. Therefore, you are not carrying around extra weight all day.

Water retention may cause the body to perform improperly. Also, increased water consumption will help the body secrete toxins. This is crucial in your healthy journey.

Dehydration - a harmful reduction in the amount of water in the body.

It is very challenging to lose weight if you are thirsty. Are you dehydrated? Watch out for the following:

✓ Dry mouth
✓ Tiredness or fatigue
✓ Sunken eyes
✓ A decrease in urination
✓ Urine that's a darker color than normal
✓ Muscle cramping
✓ Feeling dizzy or lightheaded

Action Step 7: Sugar

Pro Tip: Sugar is like a domino. This is why we can't eat just one cookie. Once you open that flood gate, it isn't easy to get back on track at times.

o **Task 1: Apply the Swap Out Method.**

1. Reduce the number of processed sugars; replace these with home-baked goods and fruit. Reserve these primarily for your Day of Indulgence. (See below)

o **Task 2: Understand How to Use All-Natural Sweeteners**

o **Task 3: Avoid Artificial Sweeteners**

o **Task 4: Practice Delayed Gratification**

Action Step 8: Day of Indulgence!

o **Task 1: Must Work Out on This Day**
o **Task 2: Plan Your Day**
o **Task 3: Don't Overdo It**
1. Be sure you only enjoy what you want

o **Task 4: Positive Reinforcement**
1. You build discipline for your mind every time you invoke delayed gratification. Eventually, your mind will adapt to this new way of living.

The key component of SAM is the caloric deficit. Understand and know your TDEE, learn to track calories, and you will know how to stay in your deficit each day effectively. You will not have to track calories forever, but this is vital for the first six weeks of your nutrition plan. Finally, I will leave you with my food debt analogy. Do you have or have you ever used a credit card? I had so much fun with my first one. I was 18 and armed with a credit card and a whopping $1000 limit. My friends and I went on a shopping spree. A few weeks later, I got a bill in the mail. I was dumbfounded or just dumb. I did not even think that far ahead. How was I going to pay this off? I tore it up and threw it in the trash, hoping it would disappear.

Well, I did not. It just kept multiplying. Years later, I had to settle and pay well over $1000. My credit score also tanked. For the next seven years, I would carry this scar. I think about food this way. I ask myself, is this choice worth the debt I will owe to my future? How is this food helping or hurting the future me I am becoming?

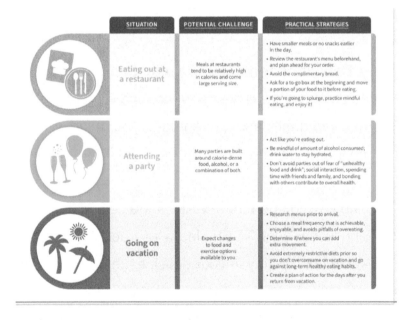

	SITUATION	POTENTIAL CHALLENGE	PRACTICAL STRATEGIES
	Eating out at a restaurant	Meals at restaurants tend to be relatively high in calories and come large serving size.	• Have smaller meals or no snacks earlier in the day. • Review the restaurant's menu beforehand, and plan ahead for your order. • Avoid the complimentary bread. • Ask for a to-go box at the beginning and move a portion of your food to it before eating. • If you're going to splurge, practice mindful eating, and enjoy it!
	Attending a party	Many parties are built around calorie-dense food, alcohol, or a combination of both.	• Act like you're eating out. • Be mindful of amount of alcohol consumed; drink water to stay hydrated. • Don't avoid parties out of fear of "unhealthy food and drink"; social interaction, spending time with friends and family, and bonding with others contribute to overall health.
	Going on vacation	Expect changes to food and exercise options available to you.	• Research menus prior to arrival. • Choose a meal frequency that is achievable, enjoyable, and avoids pitfalls of overeating. • Determine if/where you can add extra movement. • Avoid extremely restrictive diets prior so you don't overconsume on vacation and go against long-term healthy eating habits. • Create a plan of action for the days after you return from vacation.

✓ **Key points:**
➢ Consistency over perfection
➢ Where energy goes, results flow

- Take 5- when making a wrong choice, take a 5-minute break, then come back
- Walk 15 minutes- be sure your body is craving food vs. sunlight
- Make it competitive- invite family friends to play along. Who can eat the most servings of veggies in a week?
- Social comparison- Just stop it!
- Keep Premenstrual Syndrome in mind when weighing in
- Chemical restrictions- Avoid foods you can't pronounce
- Eat slow
- Spend 20-30 minutes eating each meal
- Focus on your body's language
- Character development- Are you who you say you are?

Module 5 – Fitness

"You aren't what you say; you are what you do" - Coach Mo.

<u>**Learning Objectives**</u>:

- ✓ Determine fit level
- ✓ Understand the modification checklist
- ✓ Understand how to use the cardio cheat sheet
- ✓ Recite the Importance of strength training
- ✓ Demonstrate the "Slay Body" basic moves of fitness.
- ✓ Create a weekly fitness schedule.

<u>Time: 1 hour 30 minutes or one weekly session</u>

Coach's Corner: Participants will be equipped to approach fitness at any level confidently. Participants will demonstrate proper form and have an overall foundation in functional fitness.

<u>Intro to Module 5</u>:

Are you addicted to comfort? Your comfort may be killing you, and you have no idea. We get caught up in our careers and day-to-day activities, and we often put health and fitness on the back burner. In this section, we begin to realize that our journey will not be fulfilled in its total capacity until we are whole, healthy, and healed. Can you imagine how much extra energy you would have with just a 20-minute workout per day? It is a fact that fitness activities increase our energy levels. You may not feel this at the beginning of your journey as your body is getting used to all the new movements. As you grow in your fitness journey, you will begin to get stronger and more energized, and have more precise focus along with a host of other non-scale victories. Your life will improve and enhance the work you commit towards purpose.

The non-scale achievements are significant as we do not rely totally on the scale. The scale will fluctuate up and down depending on what processes are going on inside the body. The scale can be discouraging; therefore, the scale will only be used as a measurement tool rather than the goal or benchmark. As we become more in tune with our bodies, we will not need a scale. We will know and feel when the body is in distress. Weight gain is simply a symptom of something gone awry. Maybe you are eating foods that the body does not receive well, or perhaps you are not moving your body enough. Finally, this section will continue to implement goals and milestones to move you from a temporary change to a lifestyle change.

Equipment (Optional)

✓ Resistance Bands

If you're looking to add variety to your workouts, increase your strength, and promote functional fitness, then resistance band training is a great place to start.

✓ Dumbbells

Add dumbbells to your home or office. These can be between 5-20 lbs. Add them to any functional movement.

✓ Yoga Mat

Use these mats for stretching, Yoga, Pilates, meditation, rest, and restoration.

✓ Kettlebell

Versatile equipment that can be used to follow workouts on slaybodtfitness.com

✓ Gym membership

Try out your local gym. Many gyms offer a free pass. Take advantage of the free pass to see if you enjoy the gym. Try some group classes or speak to a trainer.

✓ Foam Roller

Foam rolling is a self-myofascial release (SMR) technique. It can help relieve muscle tightness, soreness, & inflammation. And it can increase your joint range of motion. Foam rolling can be an effective tool to add to your warm-up or cooldown before and after exercise.

Action Step 1: Review the Fitness Assessment (15 min)

This will be used to customize fitness plans for participants

o **Task 1: Submit self-assessment to coach (Homework)**

o **Task 2: Submit a video of functional fitness moves (Homework)**

Coach's Corner:

Go over the assignment with the participants. Participants are encouraged to submit asap to receive a fitness plan.

Action Step 2: Slay Your Cardio- The Cardio Cheat Sheet (15 Min)

o **Task 1: Commit to 30-45 minutes of Cardio per day (MAX).** You want to burn around 200-300 calories per session.

- For sedentary workers - 3-4 days a week
- For beginners - start with two days a week
- Intermediate/advanced - 6-7 days a week

Coach's Corner: Explain why cardio is important and go over the benefits.

- Workouts will be customizable.

o **Task 2: Implement "Stress-Free Cardio" Strategies**

Don't do what you hate! There are many ways to get your cardio goal. Doing things you hate simply won't sustain. You will quit. Consistency is key; please do something you enjoy.

✓ 30 min brisk walk

Do not underestimate the power of walking. Download the Nike app or "map my fitness" and get to walking. Try creating a challenge and invite family friends to join the fun.

✓ 10K steps a day

Invest in a step tracker and commit to getting 10k steps a day. The tracker will develop discipline and increase your overall movements. Track all movements/steps. The body was made to MOVE.

✓ Dog Walking

Walking/jogging is fun for the whole family. My neighbor walks his dog at least six times per day. At least every time I go outside, I see them. The best thing about it is that the dog looks so happy.

✓ Take the kids to the park.

Many parks have walking trails. Be sure to take the kids outdoors for vitamin C and good old-fashioned fun.

✓ Active Rest Days

Be sure to plan adventurous family fun days on your rest days. This could be a day at the pool, bowling alley, golfing, skating, hiking, and so much more! Your family will be healed, and they will thank you for it.

✓ Break your workout into 2-3 parts

Hour-long workouts can seem overwhelming. Especially if you are beginning your journey or have a hectic schedule to maintain. No problem! Begin to implement 10-minute workouts into your day. This can be more effective than longer workouts. You could do 10 minutes in the morning, 10 minutes at lunchtime, and 10 minutes at night. This will free up a lot of stress and anxiety around fitness.

See www.slaybodyfitness.com/theslayacademy

✓ Bring positive energy to your workout.
✓ Visualize your goals, remember your why, and focus on the present moment

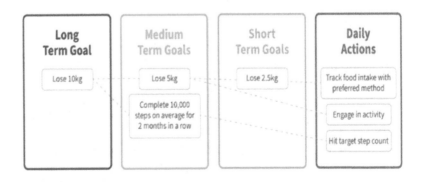

This tool will super enhance your results, do this as often and as much as possible.

> ➤ Set Goals

Set performance goals each week. For example, I want to do 40 sit-ups in 2 minutes; pushups, how many did you do in one minute? What is your goal number? Etc.

> ➤ Fasted Cardio

Coach's Corner:

Explain the steps and goals of fasted cardio. Fasted cardio is performed when your body is in a fasted state, which means it isn't digesting food. It means doing cardio on an empty stomach. This tool will super enhance your results, do this as often and as much as possible.

Action Step 3: Learn Modifications Guide

o **Task 1:** Submit and Complete the Injury Assessment and view the Modification Guide.
www.slaybodyfitness.com/theslayacademy

Action Step 4: Gain Gang! – Get Strong
Gain Muscle and lose fat at the same time. Commit to training 3-4 times a week

o **Task 1**: **If you are a novice, join a program or hire a coach**

1. For maximum results, your program should include

✓ Progressive overload

✓ Compound movements - bang for your buck

✓ Tailored overall goals

✓ Body scan

✓ 2-3 times per week - beginners

✓ 3-4 times a week - intermediate/ advanced

o **Task 2: Push it to the limit**

1. Energy - are you trying hard enough? Or are you holding back?

2. Brain Power – don't let your mind psych you out

3. Strength training will be hard and heavy; prepare mentally. I honestly believe many afflictions can be overcome by breaking the chains and limitations embedded in our minds.

Action Step 3 - Be Consistent.

What happens when you put a drop of water in a bucket? I once watched water drip into a bucket as a little girl. There was a leak in the roof and, when it would rain, my grandmother had me get a metal bucket to catch the water. I thought it was stupid to get such a big bucket for the tiny drop of water. Over time, the water filled the bucket, it overflowed, and we had to dump it. I was amazed. The systematic and consistent drops created a massive amount of water. Consistency pays off. Keep showing up and depositing your drip. Get your buckets out now, so you will be prepared for the overflow.

Action Step 4: Set your schedule

Do this monthly- *details please-* leave no room for guessing.

o **Task 1 - Plan the time to plan (20 min.)**
  - ✓ What days will you meal prep? Add this to your calendar or habit tracker.
  - ✓ What day will you do cardio?
  - ✓ What days are designated for strength training?

Action Step 5: KISS!

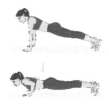

o **Task 1: See the "5 basic moves" diagram**

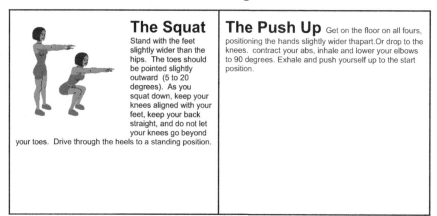

The Squat Stand with the feet slightly wider than the hips. The toes should be pointed slightly outward (5 to 20 degrees). As you squat down, keep your knees aligned with your feet, keep your back straight, and do not let your knees go beyond your toes. Drive through the heels to a standing position.

The Push Up Get on the floor on all fours, positioning the hands slightly wider thapart.Or drop to the knees. contract your abs, inhale and lower your elbows to 90 degrees. Exhale and push yourself up to the start position.

The Plank (high/Low) Place

hands directly under the shoulders. Spread the fingers wide (you can leave your knees down). Parallel your legs to the ceiling; engage the thighs. Tuck hip bones forward toward your belly to increase your abdominal and glute engagement. Stack your heels over the ball-mounts of your feet to avoid strain on the knees.

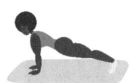

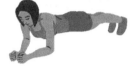

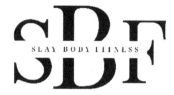

Visit

www.slaybodyfitness.com/theslayacademy

for customized or sample fitness plans.

The Lunge Stand tall

with feet shoulder width apart. Take a large step forward ensuring the heel of the foot hits first. Lower the body until the right thigh is parallel to the floor and the right shin is vertical. Be sure the knee doesn't go past the right toe. Repeat on each side.

The Dumbbell Row Grab a set of

dumbbells, bend the torso forward and keep

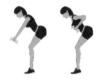

the knees slightly bent. Pull the dumbbells toward the waistline, while squeezing the shoulder blades. Slowly lower the weights to the starting position. (1-second pull, 1-second pause, 2 second down count) Repeat

Coach's Corner: Form is critical - we will evaluate your form over the next three weeks. Encourage participants to record themselves making each move. (Homework)

Exercise increases performance, endurance, and strength; and weight loss is a side effect. Exercising just for weight loss will not sustain you. Your focus would be incorrect. I once left the gym after a 2–3-hour workout. I felt discouraged because I did not feel the results of the workout. Be careful of this. Exercise can trigger the process that will lead to a total life transformation. If you switch your focus to strength building, flexibility, and endurance, your performance will continue to grow. Don't be distracted by weight loss; the focus here is growth.

✓ **Key points-**

• Start small and gradually build – doing too much too soon will overwhelm you.
• Fail to plan = plan to fail - preparation is vital. You are more likely to eat well and exercise if you plan it.
• Don't skip the Warmup
• Don't skip the cooldown
• Weekly Weigh-in (Optional) (upload stats to tracking app or excel tracker)
• Measurements - (Mandatory) – arms, legs, waist, neck, chest

Module 6 - Rest Recovery Relaxation (RRR) and sleep

Learning Objectives:

- ✓ Promote restoration and healing
- ✓ Learn how to fuel the soul
- ✓ Learn De-stress techniques
- ✓ Explore the importance of sleep
- ✓ Understand why Self-Care is vital
- ✓ Engineer the perfect night's sleep

Time: 30 minutes

Coach's Corner: Here, we focus on Healing the mind, body, and soul. We will discuss different modes and practices that participants can add to their daily schedules.

The process of weight loss and recovery happens at rest. As we begin to move our bodies more frequently, we cause some wear and tear. However, our bodies are magical. They have the power to heal themselves if we allow them to rest. More specifically, to sleep. Healing and weight loss happen in the deepest sleep. Our bodies have a similar makeup to the earth. Even the Creator of this good earth rested on the 7th day. Here we will begin to explore ways to restore healing.

Action Step 1: Earn Your Rest Day.

Be sure to complete all scheduled workouts/activities.

Commit to completing the schedule no matter what!

Action Step 2: Stress Management

- Yoga is a physiological practice that will help handle stress
- Eliminate outside noise
- Use oil diffusers
- Meditate
- Talk Therapy
- Say "no" and mean it
- Spend time in nature
- Date yourself
- Phone a friend
- Commit to managing stress

Action Step 3: Self-care

- Implement YOU time
- Spend some time alone to recharge
- Organize a spa day
- Indulge in a massage
- Don't skip your pedicure
- Be sure to put self-care on the calendar with your other to-do items. This event must be prioritized, or it will continually be neglected.

Action Step 4: Sleep

If you're trying to lose weight, the amount of sleep you get may be just as crucial as your diet and exercise. Unfortunately, many people aren't getting enough sleep. Sleep may be the missing factor for many people who have difficulty losing weight.

- ➢ Lack of sleep may negatively affect hunger levels, influencing the desire to consume more calories from high fat and high sugar foods.
- ➢ The proper amount of sleep helps you control your mood and make better decisions.

o **Task 1: Enjoy at least 7-8 hours of sleep per night**

Relax, restore, and enjoy. You earned it. Be sure to reward yourself for all your strenuous efforts throughout the week. Taking regular breaks allows your body to recover and repair. It's a critical part of progress, regardless of your fitness level or sport. Otherwise, skipping rest days can lead to overtraining or burnout.

Contrary to popular belief, a rest day isn't about being lazy on the couch. It's during this time that the beneficial effects of exercise take place. Specifically, rest is essential for muscle growth. Movement creates microscopic tears in your muscle tissue. But during rest, cells called fibroblasts will repair it. This helps the tissue heal and grow, resulting in stronger muscles. Also, your muscles store carbohydrates in the form of glycogen. During exercise, your body breaks down glycogen to fuel your workout. Rest gives your body time to replenish these energy stores before your next workout. Rest increases energy and prevents fatigue, preparing your body for consistently successful movements.

✓ **Key points-**

- Incorporate 30 minutes to 1 hour of stretching per week
- Plan your "me" time
- Try to meditate at least 5 min per day
- Go to sleep and wake up skinny
- Avoid muscle fatigue and soreness

Soul-work:

List some ways you like to decompress.

_____

_____

_____

_____.

How would you be able to incorporate this into your current lifestyle?

_____

_____

_____

_____.

Module 7 – Maintenance Phase

Learning Objectives:

- ✓ Understand the importance of the maintenance phase
- ✓ Understand maintenance calories
- ✓ Learn how to build a maintenance plan

Time: 30 minutes

Coach's Corner: Participants will learn how to maintain their goal status. Participants will be equipped with the tools necessary to maintain their healthy journey.

The maintenance phase is the final phase of the process. Congratulations on reaching the ultimate milestone. This phase is often forgotten about. We achieved our goals and began to celebrate. Next thing you know, the scale is creeping back up. We worked too hard for this.

The goal is to get healthy and *stay* healthy. The last thing you want to do here is revert to your old self. You have worked too hard to create this version of yourself. It is much easier to maintain your healthy life than revert and rebuild. It only takes a simple plan. We can learn this whether you have reached the maintenance phase or not.

Action Step 1: Plan Your Phase

- 2 -3 workouts per week
- 45 to 60-minute sessions
- 2 -3 sets per exercise. Main exercises should focus on strength, power (plyometrics, Olympic lifting, core lifts [bench, squat, deadlift]), and functional mobility. Promoting overall health
- Continue a nice mix of strength training and cardio
- Maintain Proper Nutrition
- Little changes will cause weight to creep back in
- Use a scale to track weight periodically

Action Step 2: Monitor Your TDEE

- Periodically Track maintenance calories.

Type of Day	Tracking Regression	Non-Tracking Regression
Ideal Day – Low stress, standard work/college hours, nutrition is easier to practice on these days	Track calories and stay within range. Track all macronutrients.	Have a standard set number of meals. Have these meals at regular times. Have adequate protein, veggies, carbs, and fats in each meal.

Tough Day – Moderate stress, maybe some extra hours in work or college, less sleep and more cravings; overall, less time and energy to practice good nutrition.	Track calories and stay within an expanded range. Track only protein per meal. Other macronutrients are optional.	Have a standard set number of meals. Eat at times that suit best or at any time possible. Be mindful of the potential to overeat or undereat with higher stress and less sleep.
Worse Day – High stress, extra hours or commitments at work/college, poor sleep, high cravings, little to no time or energy to practice good nutrition.	Snack on higher fiber foods if the urge strikes (e.g., whole fruit). Each main meal contains protein. Cope with stress using non-food strategies, such as breathing or mindfulness exercises.	Make core food choices when and where possible. Make protein and vegetables a staple in as many meals as possible. Be mindful of the potential to overeat or undereat with higher stress and less sleep.
Really Bad, No Good, Horrible Day – The day was stressful, nutrition was not a priority, and now you feel like they are regressing.	Try not to let a discretionary food choice carry into a whole day of disinhibited eating.	Write this day off and accept that everyone has a bad day. Remember that one bad day will not make a difference but getting back on track the day after can have a positive impact. Check in to see if plans need to be significantly changed to make things easier for the days to come.

Calculate your TDEE as your weight goes up or down
Remember slight weight fluctuations are normal

Action Step 3: Maintenance Nutrition

As for nutrition, maintaining a SAM diet plan is most effective. This will help you maintain your body weight and eat at maintenance. Protein can stay the same as during your initial phase. Carbs can be reduced as training is reduced. Fats can be increased somewhat to offset the reduction in carbs and ensure hormone levels are maintained.

MAINTENANCE PHASE NUTRITIONAL GUIDELINES

Protein: 0.9g/lb. (2g/kg)

Carbs: 2.5 to 3g/kg, about half that of peak mass phase

Fat: The rest (around 1.25 to 1.5g/kg)

Note: 1kg = 2.2 pounds

Coach's Corner: What are maintenance calories? This is the calorie number needed to maintain your goal weight. This is calculated in your TDEE. Just maintain weight! If weight fluctuates by more than plus or minus a pound (0.45kg), adjust calories up or down by 250 to 500 per day.

Action Step 4: Manifestation

Throughout this book, we have been manifesting. What is Manifestation? I call it the secret weapon. According to our friends at Merriam-Webster, manifestation is the act or process of making something evident. Manifestation is the transmutation of thought into its physical equivalent. It's the process of taking an idea, a dream, a goal, or a vision and taking the necessary action steps to make it a reality. Anything you can daydream about; you can create in your life. The Latin root of "manifestation" is "manifestare" which means "make public." What does it mean to 'manifest something'? In this case, manifestation is bringing the things you focus on to your physical reality through thoughts, feelings, and beliefs. In many ways, yes. But that doesn't mean you need to hold a specific set of beliefs to be able to manifest. Learning how to manifest what you want is much easier than you think. Use your Power, your Gut, your instinct to direct you. Not your emotions. The power is within you, you do not have to do this alone, you just need to do your part.

- o **Task 1: How to Manifest What You Want**
  - ✓ Believe in yourself – choose to pursue it.
  - ✓ Creative visualization is a great way to initiate this becoming.
  - ✓ Visualize yourself believing in yourself.
  - ✓ Acknowledge that you are capable

- o **Task 2: Create an Action Plan**
  - ✓ Write the plan
  - ✓ Work the plan
  - ✓ Have expectation

o **Task 3: Act**

  ✓ Write down your goals, both long and short-term.
  ✓ Practice breathing and meditation.
  ✓ Stay physically active, move your body.
  ✓ Tell yourself, everyone you know, and even strangers, what it is that you intend to accomplish.
  ✓ Keep a gratitude journal and write in it daily.
  ✓ Focus on the positive
  ✓ Visualize
  ✓ What you can visualize in your mind, you can hold in your hands. So, get to work! You have 'manifesting' to do!"

The next step is to be mindful of—and thankful for—what you receive.

- Stay humble and grateful

- Upgrade your beliefs

- And let go of any resistance and limiting beliefs.

- Check your energy

- Be flexible

- Trust the process

- Come in expectation

If you think it, feel it, have faith in it with intent and positivity, it will become. There's a lot of people who are eager to see instant results. Even though manifesting something quickly is possible, you must remember that the universe's plan may be different than what you have in mind. Despite all these tactics you can use to stay positive and accomplish what you want in life, the most important one can be summed up in three words: Don't give up! Quitting won't get you any closer to your goals, nor will it put you in a positive headspace. Use this guide to keep moving forward no matter how difficult life can be. Quitting too soon can cause you to miss your purpose in life, and those assigned to your purpose. Everything about you is valuable.

Slay Body Fitness

Individual Healthy Development Plan

Guide to Your Whole Health

(Coach's Version)

Individual Development Plan –

IDP is a *process* the client directs, under your guidance and support, in partnership with their mentor, to enhance their professional growth by:

- *Identifying and pursuing their personal goals for a new healthy lifestyle*

- *Setting goals to learn or improve habits they will need to maintain a healthy future*

- *Identifying their strengths, talents and passions and planning ways to use and enhance their lifestyle*

As a part of the IDHP, the Client will identify health goals that matter to them, determine what experiences, skills and behaviors will help them achieve those goals and then create a plan of action to achieve their goals. They will work with you to evaluate areas where they are already creating healthy habits and expound on that. We can succeed together.

This booklet explains your role in supporting and guiding a client's Healthy Lifestyle transformation, personal development and provides you with tools to help launch their Individual Healthy Development Plan.

Ingredients for Personal Development

Coach's Role

1. Listen to what your client is great at, where they want to be, and what they love doing and what energizes them. Provide insights into what physical activities align with what they already love. Explain how the client's current strengths can benefit the journey. Provide information to the client about areas they should improve upon first.

Getting Started – *A Step-By-Step Guide to the IHDP Process*

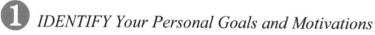 *IDENTIFY Your Personal Goals and Motivations*

- What motivates and energizes you?
- What kinds of personal and professional goals do you want in the future?
- Are their opportunities in your current daily schedule that will help you find time to develop and grow?
- Do your motivations and the needs strongly align?
- What do you want to learn...prepare for?
- Note your goals and motivations on the IHDP Conversation Tool which follows.

② *DETERMINE Your Talents/Strengths and Development Opportunities*

- What are your talents/strengths?
- What are your passions, what do you love doing?
- What are your areas to improve, or new areas to learn?
- How can we align your goals to be consistent with your talents, strengths & development needs?

③ *PLAN Your Focused IHDP Objectives and Action Steps*

- Considering your current life situation and future aspirations, where should you focus your development? What will your objectives be for this IHDP?
- Which of your strengths/talents will you use more often, or expand?
- What Healthy Transformations are important for you to focus on?
- What SMART action steps will you take to achieve your IHDP?

④ *MEET with Your Coach;*

Schedule a one-hour meeting with your client to discuss your draft IHDP.

- Prepare by reading through the "Meet with Your Client" section of this guide.
- Bring the notes you created in Step 3 to the meeting.
- Meet with your Client again to discuss and refine your individual health development plan.
- Schedule a 30-minute follow up meeting with your client to discuss the IHDP, make any changes if needed for final approval.

5 *ACT On Your Plan*

- Complete an IHDP form to finalize the plan and give a copy to your client.
- Have clients plan the IHDP deadlines into their calendar.
- Partner with your client to make the plan work.
- Schedule monthly follow up meetings with your client to check on their progress.
- Act on the plan and assume ownership.

Meet with Your Coach

The IHDP Meeting

Individual Healthy Development Planning is a partnership, a joint effort, *led* by the client and *supported* and developed by the Mentor/Coach. The plan begins to come alive during the IHDP meeting. In this first meeting, the client and coach discuss and refine the ideas they have prepared before the meeting, and talk about development within the current job, and possibilities for future career development after the client shares areas of interest, passions, talents, and long-term goals.

BEFORE & AFTER

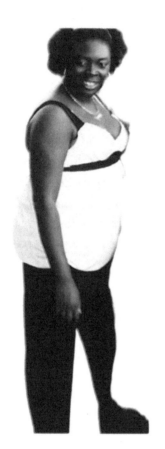 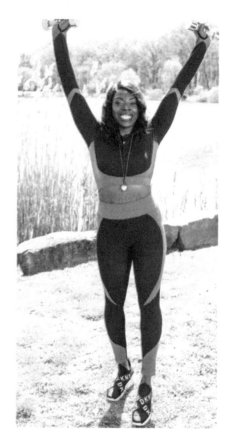

DEDICATION

This book is dedicated to the memory of my loving parents, Susie and Willie Rouse who taught me how to love.

Made in the USA
Columbia, SC
23 September 2022

67477508R00057